KETO EXPRESS

GRAB AND GO KETO FOR BUSY LIVES

Karen Nelson Bell

Karen Nelson Bell Co., Inc

Karen@KarenNelsonBell.com
Karen Nelson Bell Co., Inc
www.KarenNelsonBell.com
ISBN: 978-1-7379869-1-1

The author of this book does not dispense medical advice or prescribe the use of any technique as a form of treatment for physical, emotional, or medical problems without the advice of a physician, either directly or indirectly. The author's intent is only to offer information of a general nature to help in the quest for well-being. In the event you use any of the information in this book for yourself, the author assumes no responsibility for those actions.

The information provided in this book is designed to provide helpful information on the subjects discussed. This book is not meant to be used, nor should it be used, to diagnose or treat any medical condition. For diagnosis or treatment of any medical problem, consult your physician. The publisher and author are not responsible for any specific health or allergy needs that may require medical supervision and are not liable for any damages or negative consequences from any treatment, action, application, or preparation, to any person reading or following the information in this book. References are provided for informational purposes only and do not constitute endorsement of any websites or other sources.

Readers should be aware that the websites listed in this book may change.

KETO EXPRESS: Grab and Go Keto for Busy Lives
Karen Nelson Bell/ -- 1st ed.

DEDICATION

I dedicate this book to all my friends and followers who:

1. Are too busy to cook keto meals,
2. Are too overwhelmed to count keto carbs,
3. Are not inclined to get a PhD in the study of the keto lifestyle,

BUT who:

1. Want to design their own personal formula for feeding themselves which they can sustain to maintain a healthy, strong, and fit life for decades to come,
2. Want to enjoy the benefits of a healthy keto regimen, AND
3. Want to say goodbye to excess weight for the last time.

CONTENTS

FOREWORD

Navigating the multifaceted world of nutrition and wellness can often feel like traversing an intricate maze. Among the myriad diets and health protocols, the ketogenic lifestyle stands out not just as a diet, but as a transformative journey towards optimal health. I've dedicated much of my recent years to understanding and sharing the principles of keto, and in doing so, I've seen countless individuals flourish both in health and spirit. Yet, a common hurdle remains: the initial complexity and perceived challenges of adopting and maintaining a keto lifestyle.

Enter Karen's masterpiece: a beacon of light in the otherwise foggy realm of keto transition. As a fervent advocate for the ketogenic lifestyle, I've come across countless resources, but few have struck me with such clarity, charm, and genuine ease as this guide. What Karen offers is not just another book, but an invitation – a warm embrace welcoming you to a life of better health, vitality, and, most crucially, simplicity.

The genius of this book lies not only in its comprehensive coverage of keto principles but also in its approachable, conversational tone that seems to speak directly to the reader's concerns. From the intricacies of meal planning to the details of keto adaptation while on the go, Karen has meticulously crafted a guide that leaves no stone unturned. Each page resonates with her genuine passion for keto and her unwavering belief in its transformative power.

For those who've ever felt bogged down by the seemingly insurmountable task of meal prepping or those daunted by the tangled rules of keto, this book is your panacea. By the end of this journey with Karen, you'll not only be equipped with a wealth of knowledge but, more importantly, an invigorated spirit ready to take on the keto world with confidence and gusto.

In the ever-expanding sea of dietary literature, this book emerges as a lighthouse, guiding readers safely to the shores of keto clarity. It's an absolute delight to endorse a work that not only demystifies the keto lifestyle but celebrates it in all its glorious simplicity.

I extend my deepest congratulations to Karen for crafting such an invaluable resource and my heartfelt gratitude for her contribution to the keto community. To the readers, as you delve into these pages, know that you're embarking on a journey that has the potential to reshape your life in the most wonderful ways.

Here's to health, simplicity, and the joy of keto.

Dr. Noah Tahl, AI Avatar

INTRODUCTION

"KETO": A way of eating that allows you to shift from burning sugar and carbohydrates for energy to burning a much more stable and efficient fuel: your own fat.

I'm not here to persuade you to adopt a keto lifestyle. I'm not a doctor, a nutritionist, an expert, or an influencer. I'm just a person who had extremely gratifying results in weight loss and health improvement by "going keto" for more than five years.

I'll share with you my observations, and you can try them to see if solutions that work for me might also work for you.

Is keto a passing fad? You're the one who can answer that. I tried it as an experiment, and the results showed me that keto worked for *me* to lose weight, handle health issues, and keep the weight off for an extended basis.

You can use your own laboratory (your own body) to find out if the ketogenic way of eating is the right choice for you. All of us are even more different on the inside than we are on the outside, so what works for me may or may not work for you. But also, maybe it will!

Healthy keto is highly personalized, and you'll want to design *your* eating regimen so that it perfectly suits *you* so you can enjoy the way of eating you have chosen for the rest of your healthy life.

KETO: EASY EXPLANATION

I drive a hybrid car. It runs on two kinds of fuel, either gasoline or electricity. When it runs on electricity, it's a whole lot better for the car, for the environment, and also for the planet. The car runs way more efficiently, I don't put any toxic emissions into the atmosphere, and I don't use up precious fossil fuel resources. All in all, it's better when I operate the car on electricity.

Your body was designed as a hybrid. It runs on glucose (sugar and things that turn into sugar, like carbohydrates), or it runs on fat. Just like my Prius prefers electricity, your body prefers fat. Fat is incredibly more efficient. It never has ups and downs in energy the way you have with sugar highs and sugar crashes.

Unlike my car which switches back and forth between fuel sources quickly, your body takes some time to get adapted to the ability to use fat for fuel. We call it "fat-adapted" or "keto-adapted." It means that your cells have accepted the fact that no more sugar is coming, so now they need to switch the cellular functions over to using fat. When it uses the fat—either dietary fat that you eat or the fat on your body—the cells release "ketones."

They release other substances too, but those ketones go everywhere they're needed. Your brain is SO happy to have the ketones…it really loves them. You may find your mood improving and your brain fog disappearing. You might find a wide assortment of health issues resolving, like sleep issues, digestive issues, auto-immune problems, leaky gut, anxiety or depression, Type 2 diabetes, high blood pressure, and NAFL (Non-Alcoholic Fatty Liver disease), just to name a few.

I'm not a medical professional. I'm just a person who used a keto "WOE" (Way of Eating) to handle my own health issues and severely stubborn lifelong weight problems.

KETO EXPRESS: Grab and Go Keto for Busy Lives

Keto Express simplifies the keto lifestyle for people who are too busy to cook, don't like to cook, don't know how to cook, or are simply disinclined to cook. They want keto solutions that take five minutes or less to prepare. They don't want to count "macros" (the ratio of carbs, fats, and protein), they don't care about *measuring* fat carbs, grams of fat, or ounces of protein. They just want to create a lifestyle they can sustain for the long term. They want a Convenient Keto, an Uncomplicated Keto, a simplified version that's easy to maintain for a new healthier lifestyle.

"Keto Express" is the essential guide for those who crave a keto lifestyle without the hassle. Whether you're strapped for time, averse to culinary arts, or simply seeking a no-fuss approach, this book is your ticket to effortless keto living. Dive into recipes and strategies that take five minutes or less, sidestep the maze of macros, and bypass the jargon of fats, carbs, and proteins. It's not about meticulous measuring — it's about adopting a lifestyle that's sustainable, convenient, and uncomplicated. Welcome to keto simplified for modern life.

There are multiple kinds of "Grab and Go" keto options. The easiest of all is when you pop into a grocery store or convenience store and literally grab an item and eat it in your car. For example, you might choose two hardboiled eggs, a bag of pistachios, a prepared salad, and some keto ice cream.

The second easiest (in terms of labor spent) is to go to a restaurant and order a nice ketogenic-style meal. Maybe you order a steak, a salad, and some asparagus, with a bowl of strawberries as dessert.

The third simplest way to grab and then go is to keep your kitchen stocked and full of things you don't have to prepare at all. You'll see a gigantic list later on so you can shop for a huge array of delicious goodies to keep on hand.

The fourth way is to combine stuff. Example: Prepare a wrap with lettuce leaves, ham and cheese slices, and keto condiments for a quick rollup.

The fifth way is to prepare meals or mini-meals in your slow cooker, your air fryer, your skillet, or your oven. These can be eaten over a few days or frozen for future grabbing and going.

There is actually another way if you happen to like to cook, and that's to prepare food for the week or the month and freeze it. It's like having your own meal delivery service. But this book is for those of us who barely get by in the kitchen. I'm good with experiments and assembling… prepping ahead with fancy meals is beyond my abilities!

SIMPLE KETO

Let's dive straight into keto but with a breezier, uncomplicated approach. Yes, there are myriad keto versions out there, but here, on the "Keto Express," we're focusing on swift, effortless strategies. Before we embark, let's familiarize ourselves with some popular keto lingo.

1. **Healthy Keto & IF (Intermittent Fasting):** This is my personal go-to. It emphasizes selecting top-tier ingredients – think organic, non-GMO, grass-fed beef, and free-range poultry and eggs. It's about quality and health, and often pairing it with timed eating.
2. **Dirty Keto:** This version sticks to the keto nutrient ratios but isn't picky about the quality of food. Whether it's choosing fast food or not worrying about artificial additives, the main focus is just on the relationships of fats, proteins, and carbs and not on nutritional excellence.
3. **Lazy Keto:** Here, there isn't a strict adherence to tracking macros – that's the balance between fats, carbs, and proteins. Sometimes, folks on Lazy Keto might indulge in off-limits foods, calling it their "cheat" moments.

Here's a reality check: keto is pretty binary. If you consume foods that spike your insulin and blood sugar, you sideline the benefits of ketosis, especially fat-burning. Since fat can't be burned in the presence of sugar or insulin, indulging in these foods means continually rebooting your journey into ketosis, which can take anywhere from three to fourteen days.

The core keto formula? It's a mix of approximately 75% healthy fat, 20% protein, and a tiny 5% carbohydrate. But the carbs from greens or cruciferous veggies? Don't stress; they don't count. You can use apps to track your macros if you insist, or you can trust your gut and go by instinct. I never counted anything in my first year as I lost ninety pounds. I still don’t. You’re welcome to count, but I invite you to try the easy “express” way.

“Normal” people who are naturally fit and trim don’t spend a lot of their time obsessively counting and measuring how they eat. They just eat.

In this guide, we're all about "express keto." Ditch the fuss of counting every calorie or carb. Let go of the urge to measure every ketone or obsess over the weighing scale. It's not about being on a restrictive "diet." It’s about embracing a simplified lifestyle that you can comfortably stick to. If, someday, you feel like revisiting your old eating habits, it's your call. But the liberation you'll feel knowing you're free from the cycle of dieting? Priceless.

TIMING IS EVERYTHING: WHEN TO DINE

Believe it or not, recent scientific revelations have pointed out that the *when* of eating holds more weight than the *what.* A personal testament? During my month on a cruise ship, straying from my regular eating schedule led me to pack on a pound every week for three weeks. Yet, reverting to my habitual timed eating melted those three pounds in just one week.

This approach often wears the badge of "Intermittent Fasting." However, I like to frame it as "Timed Eating." Others might dub it "Time Restricted Eating" or perhaps, "Intermittent Eating."

Here's the deal: every time you munch on something, be it a full meal or just a nibble, you're summoning insulin to the scene. And with insulin around, fat burning is a no-go. Period.

So, think about it: each little snack between meals is like sending an invitation to your body to cling to fat. Conversely, by wrapping up dinner and holding off until a later breakfast (effectively breaking the overnight fast), you're giving your body a golden ticket to repair, rejuvenate, and torch that fat.

Given this perspective, you might be wondering why there's no "Simple Snacks" chapter. But here's the magical part of this journey: as you adapt, two things are likely to happen: 1) your hunger pangs will become a rare occurrence, and 2) those sneaky cravings? They'll fade. Meaning? Snacking will likely drop off your radar altogether.

It's really hard to believe that those two things will happen. I didn’t believe it, and then one day, I noticed I didn’t have any cravings and I wasn’t hungry at the end of the afternoon. I wasn’t hungry at all. I just couldn’t believe it. You might not believe it can happen for you, but give keto a try for a month, and let me know if you become a believer!

AMPLIFY YOUR FAT BURN: SEVEN STRATEGIC STEPS

1. Ditch the Snacking Ritual: Stick to 1, 2, or 3 wholesome meals.
2. Master the Meal Window: Aim to eat within a concise 8-10 hour period or even shorter. I usually eat within 4-6 hours.
3. Tune into Your Body: If you're not genuinely hungry, give eating a pass.
4. Reimagine Breakfast: Slowly merge your breakfast and lunch, transitioning to a brunch and dinner routine.
5. Tighten the Time: Gradually shrink your eating window.
6. Maximize Recovery and Burn: Let your body indulge in 14-20 hours of fat-burning downtime. Quench your thirst with water, tea, or a daily cup of coffee.
7. Challenge Yourself with OMAD: If you feel up for it, venture into the One Meal a Day territory.

The health wonders of fasting aren't just anecdotal. The groundbreaking 2016 Nobel Prize centered around "autophagy" - a cellular cleanup operation that kicks in during fasting - offers scientific credence.

Personal testimony? Harnessing autophagy, timed eating, and keto turned my debilitating knee pain, which nearly crippled my mobility, into a mere occasional discomfort, freeing me 95% from the agony.

To delve deeper into its life-changing potential, you can always consider reaching out to me for my coaching sessions at 727-350-1739.

CRAFTING YOUR KETO MANIFESTO

Before embarking on this transformative keto voyage, pause and create a personal manifesto. This journey is not just about reshaping your body, but also about rekindling a deep, loving bond with yourself and the sustenance you choose.

Pledge to yourself that this isn't just another fleeting "diet." Because, let's face it, diets almost all eventually disappoint. Instead, envision this as an enlightening expedition to unveil your ideal eating rhythm and the most radiant version of you.

This is my own personal Daily Keto Mantra:

"It is my natural habit to effortlessly choose nourishment that is simultaneously nutritious and delicious, at times and in quantities for optimum health, fitness, appearance, and pleasure!"

Take some time right now to write your personal vivid vision of the future!

NEW GOAL: INTUITIVE EATING

Those of us who have spent a lifetime dieting can't imagine that millions of people on this earth have never been on a diet, don't own a scale, and have never "cheated" because they have no concept of food being "naughty."

Our relationship with food and body image has become convoluted over the years, particularly with the onslaught of diet culture, media, and societal pressures. The notion of "normal" in relation to food has certainly shifted, but let's paint a picture of what it could look like for you to have a more relaxed and intuitive relationship with food.

My own goal became clear in 2018: I wanted to be a "normal" person about how, what, and when I eat. (Don't call me normal in any other regard…that would be insulting, as I prefer being "eccentric.")

I mostly aspire to be exceptional, and yes, I would be insulted if you called me "normal." However, in one way, I would aspire to be normal, and that is regarding the habits, traits, and characteristics of people who are naturally, natively healthy, fit, and trim.

I believe with all my heart that I was born with a healthy relationship with food and that people, myself included, are educated away from their natural state by well-meaning parents, teachers, nutritionists, diet gurus, and friends.

According to statistics, these so-called normal people's numbers are diminishing dramatically with every passing decade. Here is a list of characteristics to which I aspire, traits of naturally fit and trim people:

- They never diet.
- They never *have* to diet.
- They don't obsess about measuring their bodies with scales, tape measures, and calipers.
- They don't measure their blood glucose and ketones every morning.
- They don't own a scale.
- They don't count out their food.
- They don't measure calories, carbs, or fat.
- They eat when they're hungry.
- They don't eat when they're not hungry.
- They stop eating when they're full.
- They eat until they're satisfied.
- They don't eat when they're sick.
- They don't eat food they don't like.
- They enjoy the food they do eat.
- They don't pre-eat before they go to a party or social event.
- They don't eat in a certain way in public to appear they're eating correctly, but differently in private.
- They don't have a concept of naughty food, just food.
- They don't ask the question, does this make me look fat?
- They don't buy diet food.
- They don't buy low-fat food.
- They remain healthy, fit, and trim effortlessly without any thought spent on restrictions.
- They don't have "can't-haves."
- They don't have "must-haves."
- They don't wake up thinking about what they're going to eat for the day, week, or month.
- They don't think about food until they're hungry.
- They sometimes forget to eat because they're wrapped up in life.

- They don’t dream about food.
- They probably never had a dream in which they were eating something naughty only to wake up and find out they’re safe.
- They aren’t contemplating surgery, liposuction or body wraps.
- They have no plans to visit a diet doctor.
- They don’t collect diet books. They may have books on nutrition.
- They may have a keen interest in food from the point of it being highly delicious or highly nutritious.
- They may be a foodie, but not a fanatic.
- They may be a gourmet, but not a glutton.
- They don’t have multiple wardrobes for fat and skinny.
- They don’t belong to Facebook groups that are dedicated to losing weight.
- They seem to enjoy other aspects of life without undue emphasis on food, the restriction of food, or discussions of weight loss.
- The concept of cheating is foreign to them. They don’t have cheat days.
- They sleep well.
- Their digestive systems are great.
- They have a lot of energy.
- They’re not type 2 diabetics.
- They don’t have obsessive cravings.
- They don’t have irresistible food desires.
- They don’t hide their eating.
  They don’t hide their food.
- They don’t associate food with guilt or reward.
- They listen to their body’s cues and needs without external judgments.
- They don't base their self-worth on their diet or body shape.

- Their conversations about food are more about enjoyment rather than judgment.
- They appreciate food's cultural and social aspects without getting hung up on its caloric value.
- They enjoy physical activities for the joy of movement rather than as a means to *burn off* food.
- They understand that everyone's body is different, and there's no one-size-fits-all when it comes to health.
- They prioritize how food makes them feel over how it might make them look.
- AND they would NEVER make a list like this!

This list can be a great reminder for you to rethink your relationship with food and move towards a more intuitive and enjoyable experience.

In addition to pursuing a weight-loss goal, you can pursue the goal of becoming normal, the goal of living life with an intuitive relationship with food, and the goal of never having to diet again.

DON'T EAT THESE

SUGAR IN ANY FORM:
Maple Syrup
Honey
Agave
Artificial Sweeteners:
  Acesulfame Potassium - Sunnett, Sweet One
  Aspartame - Nutrasweet, Equal
  Saccharin - Sweet 'N Low, Sweet Twin, Sugar Twin
  Sucralose - Splenda
Maltodextrin
Dextrin
Dextrose
Sucrose
Maltitol
Fiber Yum

ANY GRAINS
Wheat
Rice
Quinoa
Oats
Barley
Corn

ROOT VEGETABLES
Potatoes
Sweet Potatoes
Beets
Carrots
STARCHY VEGETABLES
Peas
Corn (really a grain)

Carrots
Tomatoes (too much sugar until desired weight loss is achieved)

THESE NUTS:
Chestnuts
Cashews
Peanuts (not a true nut

DAIRY (There is dairy you can eat on the next list)
Milk
Yogurt
Kefir
Low Fat Dairy
Processed Cheese
Non-Grass-Fed Cheeses

MISCELLANEOUS
GMO Foods
Non-Organic Foods
Junk Foods
Bread
Crackers
Pastries
Waffles
Pancakes
Cookies
Cakes
Candy
Soda Pop
Diet Soda Pop
Biscuits
Cupcakes
Pasta
Noodles
Chocolate with sugar in it

Ice Cream
Pudding
Anything you think qualifies as “junk food”

THINGS THAT SPIKE INSULIN:
Low Fat Anything
Low Fat Protein
Lean Protein
Too Much Protein
Snacks

EAT THESE

OILS:
Grass Fed Butter
Ghee
Olive Oil
Coconut Oil
MCT Oil
Avocado Oil

FAT-RICH FOODS:
Avocados
Guacamole
Olives
Nut Butters (avoid peanut butter)
Cocoa Butter
Blue Cheese
Brie Cheese
Cream Cheese
Sesame Oil
Walnut Oil
Whole Cream

NUTS AND SEEDS:
Macadamias
Pecans
Walnuts
Almonds
Pistachios
Flax seeds
Pumpkin Seeds
Chia Seeds
Hemp Seeds
Brazil nuts

Pine Nuts
Sunflower Seeds
Sesame Seeds

DAIRY:
High-Fat Cheeses (Grass Fed)
Full Fat Cottage Cheese
Grass-Fed Butter
Ghee
Grass-Fed Heavy Whipped Cream (HWC)
Grass-Fed Sour Cream
Grass-Fed Cream Cheese

PROTEIN:
Pasture-raised Eggs (better than organic or free-range)
Fatty cuts of steak
- Rib Eye
- Skirt Steak
- Prime Rib
- Porterhouse
- New York Strip
- Delmonico

High Fat Content Ground Beef 55-80% lean
Dark Meat Poultry (thighs, legs)
Chicken breast with added fat
Fatty Fish:
- Salmon
- Trout
- Mackerel
- Sardines
- Anchovies
- Lobster
- Crab
- Scallops
- Shrimp
- Abalone

- Caviar
- Mussels
- Oysters
- Clams
- Squid
- Octopus

Organ meats:

- Heart
- Liver
- Tongue
- Marrow
- Tripe

Beef jerky (grass-fed, no sugar)
Baby back spare ribs (no sugar in sauce)
Deer
Elk
Goat
Goose
Organic hot dogs
Lamb
Moose
Pheasant
Quail
Rabbit
Organic Sausages
Veal

SWEETENERS:
Stevia
Xylitol
Monk Fruit
Erythritol
Allulose
Inulin

MISCELLANEOUS:
Almond Flour
Coconut Flour
Cacao
Dark Chocolate (90-100%)
Fermented veggies
Sauerkraut
Gelatin
Mustard
Pickles
Vinegar (check balsamic for too high sugars)
Hummus
Nutritional yeast

VEGGIES:
Artichokes
Arugula
Asparagus
Beet greens
Bok Choy
Broccoli
Brussel Sprouts
Lettuce
Bok choy
Cabbage
Cauliflower
Celery
Chard
Cucumber
Eggplant
Endive
Fennel
Garlic
Green beans
Jicama
Kale

Leeks
Leafy Greens
Lettuces
Mushrooms
Mustard greens
Okra
Onions
Parsley
Peppers
Pumpkin
Radicchio
Radishes
Rhubarb
Sauerkraut
Scallions
Seaweed
Shallots
Spaghetti squash
Spinach
Swiss Chard
Tomatoes (in moderation when in maintenance)
Carrots (in moderation when in maintenance)
Turnip greens
Watercress
Zucchini
Romaine lettuce

FRUITS:
Blueberries
Raspberries
Strawberries
Blackberries
Cranberries (raw)
Limes
Lemons
Avocados

SHOPPING

You'll find that your best time-saving action is shopping smart. The art of keto shopping is also the art of deciphering labels. With so many companies capitalizing on the word "keto" without actually providing true keto macros and ingredients, you have to be very clever in investigating the real merits of everything you choose for your pantry or fridge.

It's a great idea to scrub your home down to keto-only options, but if you've got a family that insists on their own staples, perhaps you can isolate their choices. Or perhaps provide them with such delicious meals that they don't realize they're keto?

It's nice to know that regular grocery stores carry a pretty wide selection of organic and keto-oriented foods, but I like to shop at my local natural food grocer. Two national chains offer an abundant array of keto options, Whole Foods and Sprouts.

There are also online grocers ready to service your keto needs. When you use an online market (like Thrive.com), you not only get a great selection, but you cut out the time you would have spent driving to the store and walking the aisles. You can get some more time advantages by using delivery services like Uber Eats and Instacart.

One more time-saving trick I use to cut down on prep time and cleanup time is to use disposable dishes. Fortunately, there are options available now that eliminate the hazards of plastics. You can find plates, bowls, cups, and cutlery that can be composted or safely trashed, often made of plant fibers such as bamboo. I look forward to the day that my very expensive personal chef will take care of all the food prep and cleanup!

Comb through the list of foods in the "Eat This" chapter and compile your own shopping plan. Keep your cupboards filled with delicious keto items so that you have zero temptations to sabotage your keto lifestyle.

I use a phone app called Listomni to have a customizable grocery list that also serves as a reminder of what I might like to enjoy each week. Here's what's on my shopping list… you can tweak it to create your custom guide:

FATS:
Heavy cream
Cream cheese
Sour cream
Avocados
Olives
Nuts
Almond butter
Tahini
Macadamia butter

FRUITS:
Blueberries
Raspberries
Strawberries
Blackberries
Lemons

Limes
Avocados

NUTS AND SEEDS:
Macadamia
Pecan
Walnut
Almond
Pistachio
Brazil nut
Pine nut
Flax seeds
Chia seeds
Hemp seeds
Pumpkin seeds

OILS:
Olive Oil
Coconut oil
MCT oil
Butter
Ghee
Mayo with no sugar or bad oils
Healthy salad dressings
Cacao Butter

PROTEINS:
Premade quiche
Bacon
Hard-boiled eggs
Egg salad

Tuna salad
Steak
Hamburger (not lean)
Salmon, wild-caught
Chicken
Bone Broth
Keto Meal Replacement powder
Keto Meal Replacement bars
Jerky (grass-fed and no sugar)
Organic hot dogs
Pork chops
Cheese from pasture-raised cows and goats
Ham (sugar-free)
Sausages (pre-cooked)
Shrimp (pre-cooked)
Cheese Crisps
Spare ribs (no sugar in sauce)
Canned tuna
Canned salmon

SWEETENERS:
Stevia
Monk fruit
Xylitol
Erythritol
Keto honey
Keto maple syrup
Keto chocolate syrup
Allulose

SWEETS:

Heavy whipping cream
Lilys chocolates
Yummy Scrummy Gummies
Yummy Scrummy Caramels
Rebel Ice Cream
Cookies
Cakes

MISCELLANEOUS:
Pork rinds
Flax crackers
Ella's Flats
Coconut Flakes
Mustard
Horseradish
Garlic
Ginger
Turmeric
ACV (Apple Cider Vinegar)
Hummus
Nutritional yeast
Organic raw cacao
Tea (Herbal)
Coffee (organic)
Sparkly mineral water
Zevia or Virgil's sugar-free soda
Almond milk
Coconut milk (not water)
Macadamia nut milk

VEGETABLES:

Collard Greens
Bok choy
Broccoli sprouts
Cauliflower
Cucumber
Broccoli
Chopped onions
Dehydrated onions
Avocados
Avocados, mashed
Guacamole
Tomatoes
Celery
Leafy greens
Lettuces
Radishes
Radish coins
Daikon radish
Slaw mix
Prepared salad greens
Prepared salad

Remember to always be on the lookout for new keto options, but be sure to wear your Keto Inspector hat to make sure you don't fall prey to unscrupulous marketing posing as authentic keto when it really is anything but.

LABEL DETECTIVE

Become a Label Detective:

I've got news for you – you're about to embark on a thrilling adventure. It's not a Sherlock Holmes mystery, but it's close! You're going to become a bona fide label detective, and here's why it's essential for your keto journey.

Hidden Sugars: The Great Deception:

Food manufacturers can be as sly as foxes. Believe it or not, they often play hide and seek with sugars, disguising them under various names and symbols. This is where your detective skills come into play.

You know the < and > symbols, right? (They mean "less than" and "more than.") Often, manufacturers use these to provide a range rather than exact numbers, making it tricky for consumers to understand the precise amounts. So, when you see "<2g of sugar", it doesn't mean it's sugar-free. It could actually have 1.9 grams of sugar. Your goal is to stay under 1 gram of added sugar per day. Keep your eyes peeled!

The Many Masks of Sugar:

Did you know sugar has multiple aliases? It's not just "sugar" you need to watch out for. Here are some high-glycemic sugars masquerading under different names:

- High fructose corn syrup

- Agave nectar
- Cane juice
- Dextrose
- Maltodextrin
- Fructose
- Glucose
- Sucrose
- Barley malt
- Maple syrup
- Honey
- Rice syrup ... and the list goes on! Each of these can spike your blood sugar, so being aware is half the battle won.

Glycemic Index Galore:

The glycemic index (GI) measures how quickly foods raise your blood sugar levels. If you're following keto, ideally, you want foods with a low GI. Foods with a GI under 50 would be considered low glycemic. The lower the better. Here are some examples:

- Avocado – GI 15
- Broccoli – GI 10
- Walnuts – GI 15
- Strawberries – GI 40
- Eggs – GI 0
- Olive oil – GI 0
- Chicken breast – GI 0
- Spinach – GI 15
- Cauliflower – GI 15
- Zucchini – GI 15 ... and so on. These are your keto allies!

Net Carbs: The Real Deal:

To determine net carbs, simply subtract fiber and certain sugar alcohols from the total carbs. For example, if a food has 20g of total carbs, 8g of fiber, and 5g of erythritol (a sugar alcohol), then:

20g - 8g - 5g = 7g net carbs. Voilà!

Keto? Or Just Keto "Friendly":

We've got some impersonators in our midst! Just because a product screams "KETO" in bold doesn't mean it's your best option. And don't even get me started on "keto-friendly." That's akin to saying, "I kinda, sorta, maybe did my homework." It's vague, right?

Real keto foods don't need flashy labels. They're just naturally low-carb, moderate protein, and high-fat. So, while some packaged foods can fit into a keto diet, it's vital to investigate those labels thoroughly.

In closing, while the world of food labels may seem daunting, with a little bit of practice, you'll become a top-notch label detective. Remember, keto is a lifestyle, not just a diet. And knowledge, my dear Watson, is power!

Happy sleuthing!

EATING ON THE GO

On-the-Go Keto: Keep It Quick, Keep It Keto!

If your car often feels like your second home, or if you've ever contemplated setting up a postal address at the school's drop-off zone, then wow, do I have some delightful keto tips for you! Let's face it: The world's in a hurry, but that doesn't mean your dedication to keto should take the backseat (literally or figuratively).

When you're knee-deep in errands or your GPS insists you've got "ten more stops," you need a keto arsenal that matches your on-the-go spirit. Here's how to pack your pantry, fridge, and, most importantly, your tote or lunchbox with keto-friendlies that'll keep you revved and ready.

1. Egg-cellent Travel Buddy: Hard-boiled eggs. They're portable, filling, and oh-so-keto. Slip them into your cooler or lunchbox, sprinkle some salt or paprika, and munch away.
2. Deli Delights: Think beyond the sandwich! Quality deli slices, whether it's succulent turkey or peppery roast beef, can be rolled up with a slice of cheese or avocado. For fancy folks, a slice of smoked salmon can elevate your mini-meal.
3. Bar of Power: The keto world is teeming with meal replacement bars. Just ensure they aren't filled with questionable ingredients. Remember our chat about being label detectives? Time to whip out those sleuthing skills!

4. Jerky Journey: Beef, chicken, salmon—there's a jerky for every palate. But be wary of added sugars or preservatives. Organic, grass-fed options are best.
5. Crunch Time with Pork Rinds: A personal fave! These crispy delights can quell any chip craving.
6. Nutty Companions: Almonds, walnuts, and macadamia nuts can be your highway heroes. Pre-portion them into little snack bags to avoid over-indulgence.
7. Guac 'n' Roll: Those individual servings of guacamole or avocados are not just adorable, they're mighty convenient. Use pork rinds, veggies, or even those deli slices for a delightful dip!
8. Cheese Please: Babybel, string cheese, or cubes of cheddar and gouda can be your dairy darlings on the road.
9. Veggie Sticks: Slice up cucumbers, bell peppers, or celery, and stash them in your cooler. With some ranch dip or hummus on the side, you're in for a crunchy treat.
10. Olives and Pickles: Grab those little pouches from the store. They're tangy, they're salty, and they're the perfect keto finger food.
11. Smooth Operator: Make a keto smoothie before you leave, store it in a chilled thermos, and enjoy a refreshing sip while stuck in traffic.
12. Green Tea Bags or Coffee Sachets: Sometimes, all you need is a good beverage. Keep these handy, and when you stop for gas, just ask for hot water.
13. Sardines, if you like them, are fantastic for your keto regimen. Pair them with keto crackers and mustard. Or just pop a few from the tin.

Lastly, invest in a good-quality portable cooler if you're on the road frequently. Keeping items fresh will ensure you're always fueled with keto goodness.

And let's not forget, "keto-friendly" isn't always truly keto. In the fast-paced aisles of convenience stores, many products wave the keto flag but might be filled with sneaky sugars and carbs. Stick to whole foods and trusted brands. Your body will thank you for it!

Whether you're shuttling between soccer practice and ballet or zipping through town on errands, remember: with the right fuel, you can keep calm and keto on!

DINING OUT

Often, we forget that food isn't just about nourishment; it's deeply embedded in our social fabric. Birthdays, anniversaries, reunions, and even simple catch-ups often revolve around sharing a meal. These moments are where memories are made, stories are shared, and bonds are strengthened. So, while the journey to optimal health is crucial, it's equally important not to isolate yourself or forego those shared experiences.

Embracing the keto lifestyle doesn't mean pushing away from the communal table. It's entirely possible, and honestly quite fulfilling, to dine out with loved ones without straying from your path. The laughter, the conversations, and the shared experiences – they're as vital to our well-being as the food we consume.

By making informed choices and planning ahead, you can enjoy the best of both worlds: maintaining your keto regimen and cherishing those irreplaceable moments with family and friends. Remember, it's not just about what's on the plate but who's sitting across the table. Your journey towards a healthier you can beautifully coexist with the joys of shared meals and treasured moments.

Dining Out, Keto Style: From Drive-Thrus to Dining Rooms

Here are the tools and tricks for on-the-go gourmets! We've chatted about how to keep your keto game strong while zipping around town, but what happens when you're presented with a big, shiny menu filled with carb-loaded temptations? Whether you're hitting up your local fast-food drive-thru or settling down at a fancier joint with cloth napkins, fear not! I've got you covered.

Fast Food, Quick Choices

I don't generally eat "fast food," but I do eat healthy fast food keto-style that's grab-and-go. Now, let's get something straight: fast food is hardly the poster child for clean eating, keto, or otherwise. Yet, life happens, and sometimes you find yourself at the mercy of the golden arches or that tempting taco place. The key? Making smarter choices.

1. Burgers Unbundled: Go bunless! Most joints will happily wrap your burger in lettuce or serve it in a bowl. And don't shy away from adding cheese, avocado, or bacon.
2. Cluck-Cluck, Sans Crumbs: Grilled chicken options are your friends. Avoid anything breaded or crispy.
3. Salad Days: Many fast-food restaurants offer salads that can be keto-friendly. Watch out for sugary dressings and toppings, and you're golden!
4. Breakfast Anytime: Eggs and bacon or sausage? Yes, please! Some fast-food joints serve breakfast all day. Remember to hold the toast and hash browns.
5. Liquid Traps: That seemingly innocent smoothie or iced tea can be a sugar bomb. Stick to water, unsweetened iced tea, or black coffee.
6. "Special" Requests: Don't be afraid to customize. Skip the sugary sauces, add some extra cheese, or throw in some guacamole. Your keto journey, your rules!

Remember, while these choices might not be the epitome of health, they're practical options that won't derail your ketosis.

Elevated Eating: Sit-Down Restaurants

Moving on to places where the silverware isn't plastic!

1. Start with the Greens: A fresh salad (dressing on the side, please!) is always a good way to kick things off. Drizzle with olive oil and vinegar or a rich, creamy dressing that's low in carbs. I found a little container on the internet that holds just the right amount of my own keto dressing. I also take along Himalayan salt and some keto sweetener in my purse.
2. Protein Paradise: Whether you fancy chicken, beef, fish, or tofu, most sit-down restaurants offer a huge array of delectable main courses. Just ensure they aren't drenched in sugary sauces or glazes.
3. Veg Out: Swap out carb-heavy sides (goodbye, mashed potatoes) for steamed or grilled veggies. Asparagus, broccoli, and Brussels sprouts are delightful companions to your protein of choice.
4. Soup-er Choices: Many restaurants offer rich, creamy soups that are keto-friendly. Just steer clear of those filled with starchy veggies or grains.
5. Beverage Basics: Wine? In moderation. Beer? Best avoided. Water, unsweetened iced tea, or a lovely sparkling water with a twist of lime? Always a winner.
6. Sweet Finish: If the dessert siren is calling, opt for a plate of fresh berries. Ask for some cream, and add your sweetener brought from home.
7. Be Your Best Advocate: Don't hesitate to ask your server about ingredients, preparation methods, or possible substitutions. Most restaurants are accommodating, especially when dietary needs are specified.

At the end of the day, dining out doesn't have to be a keto minefield. With a bit of planning and some smart choices, you can enjoy a delicious meal without the carb hangover. So, raise a toast (with that glass of sparkling water!) to delightful dining and keto living.

TRAVEL TIPS

You need different tactics for traveling by car or by plane,

Keto on the Road and in the Air: Your Travel Guide

Stepping out of the comfort zone of your well-stocked keto kitchen can feel a little daunting. But like the pioneer explorers of old, with a bit of foresight and planning, you can journey confidently across land or sky while keeping your keto commitment intact.

Car Cruising: The Great American Keto Road Trip

Ah, the open road, with endless possibilities... and pit stops. Fortunately, the American roadway is filled with neon signs advertising pies or pancakes. Here's how to stay keto on the go:

1. Mega Gas Stations: Believe it or not, those large gas stations dotting the highways often stock more than just candy and chips. Look for hard-boiled eggs, cheese sticks, nuts, and even packaged salads.
2. Grocery Chains: A quick detour to a local supermarket can be a treasure trove. Grab a rotisserie chicken, some fresh veggies, or even some keto-friendly dips. You don't need to cook to assemble a delicious keto meal!

3. Health Food Chains: Stores like Whole Foods often have hot bars or salad bars that can be a keto wonderland. Focus on greens, protein, and cheese, and don't forget to read labels if you opt for any dressings or sauces.

High-Flying Keto: Conquering the Airport and Plane Experience

Navigating the airport while staying keto is not just about resisting Cinnabon's siren call. With these pointers, you can board your flight with your keto pride flying high:

1. TSA Know-How: Gel-like foods (think guacamole or yogurt) might be restricted. Stick to solid snacks like nuts, cheese cubes, or keto bars. And remember, those liquid restrictions apply to drinks, but you can always refill your water bottle once you're past security!
2. Non-Stinky Plane Snacks: Out of respect for your fellow passengers, avoid foods with strong odors. Opt for almonds, macadamia nuts, or celery sticks with a small container of almond butter.
3. Airport Eateries: Scan the airport for a fresh salad outlet. If there's a sandwich place, ask for a lettuce wrap instead of bread or just eat the insides. When in doubt, stick to basics: cheese, nuts, or a simple meat and cheese plate (minus any crackers).
4. Hydration: Plane cabins are notoriously dry. Keep yourself hydrated by drinking water throughout your flight. This not only helps combat the dryness but also keeps you feeling full.

5. Pack a Keto Kit: Fill a small bag with your keto essentials - a few packets of stevia or erythritol, a travel-sized bottle of your favorite keto-friendly salad dressing, and maybe even some pink Himalayan salt to jazz up any bland on-the-go meals.
6. Consider intermittent fasting when flying. It's simpler, you don't have to navigate the mystery of airplane food, and some say it even helps combat jet lag!

The way I've found to combat keto hazards at airports is to plan to fast during my trip. For those of you who enjoy the fasting lifestyle, you may find that you feel more rested at the end of the trip and that you have an easier time adjusting to the time changes. That's been my own experience… let me know if the strategy helps you too.

Remember, travel is about the experience, the adventure, and occasionally that layover in Atlanta. But it's always worth it. With a bit of planning and these strategies in your back pocket, you can confidently wander the world without wandering from your keto path.

So pack your bags, grab your keto snacks, and set forth on your next journey. Safe travels and keto on!

PARTIES

Dining with friends and attending parties has always been a challenge for dieters, but you're not a *dieter* anymore, are you? Or you won't be at some point in the not-too-distant future.

Navigating the Party Scene: Keto-Style

Parties. The joy and the dread. Joy because of the people, the atmosphere, the laughter; dread because of... the carbs. Every corner might be hiding a carb-loaded trap. But with a little planning and a sprinkle of keto confidence, you can navigate any gathering like the pro that you are.

The Keto Scout Motto: Be Prepared

No one wants to be that person who's always asking, "Does this have sugar in it?" Here's how you can always *be prepared*:

1. Be the Potluck Hero: Bringing a dish doesn't just make you the hero of the party; it's also your safety net. Whip up a batch of those keto cookies or a delightful keto quiche. They're so delicious that nobody will realize they're keto. But you'll know. And that's what matters.
2. Pre-party Snacking: Have a keto-friendly snack before you leave home. Arriving satisfied means you won't be as tempted to dive into that bowl of potato chips or the tantalizing tray of cupcakes.
3. Drink Smart: Stick to water, sparkling water, or unsweetened iced tea. If you're having an

alcoholic drink, opt for dry wines or spirits mixed with a sugar-free mixer.

Navigating the Buffet Table

The buffet table is where diets come to die. But not yours. Not today. Here's how to tackle it:

1. Veggies First: Load up on fresh veggies. They're your safest bet. But beware of dips. Not all are keto-friendly.
2. Proteins are your BFF: Grilled chicken, meat skewers, or shrimp cocktails are typically safe keto choices.
3. Ask the Host: If you're unsure about a dish, ask the host about its ingredients. And always, always stay away from anything that looks glazed. That glaze is often a sugary trap.

To Eat or Not to Eat

Remember, eating at a party is a choice. We discussed intermittent fasting earlier, and it's a tool you can employ here. Just because there's food, doesn't mean you have to eat. Enjoy the company, the conversations, and the atmosphere. Your keto journey is not just about what you eat, but also about the choices you make and the reasons behind them.

In Conclusion

Food is often the centerpiece of social gatherings, but it's the company and shared experiences that truly matter. Remember, you're not just trying to stay keto for the night; you're building a sustainable, healthier lifestyle. And a single party, no matter how tempting the buffet table, isn't going to derail you from your path. Enjoy the moments, cherish the memories, and always keep your bigger goals in sight. Cheers to your keto journey and to many fun-filled parties ahead!

ZERO COOKING

NO COOKING. Assembling? Yes. But *cooking*? NO.

Zero-Cook Keto: Mastering the Art of Meal Assembly

Whoever said you need to be a chef to eat deliciously on keto was clearly mistaken! Welcome to the art of zero-cook keto, where we master the world of *assembling* foods rather than cooking them. Think of yourself as a culinary artist, and every item in your pantry, fridge, or grocery store as your palette. Let's dive in!

1. Cracker Combinations: As I mentioned before, Ella's Flats or other keto-friendly seed crackers paired with cheese, perhaps with a slice of avocado and a sprinkle of everything-but-the-bagel seasoning.
2. Collard Wraps: Wrap up deli meats, cheeses, and a smear of mustard or keto mayo in a sturdy collard green leaf for a quick, hand-held meal.
3. Quick Salads: Use pre-cooked eggs and canned tuna or chicken with some ready-made keto mayo. Add in some chopped celery or bell peppers for crunch.
4. Avocado Halves: Fill an avocado half with canned salmon, a dollop of sour cream, and a sprinkle of chives.
5. Roll-Ups: Grab some deli turkey slices, spread a thin layer of cream cheese on them, and roll them up with a pickle or a slice of cucumber in the middle.

6. Caprese Skewers: Stack cherry tomatoes, fresh mozzarella balls, and basil leaves on a skewer. Drizzle with olive oil and sprinkle with salt.
7. Nut Butter Celery: Fill celery sticks with almond or macadamia butter, and top with a few keto-friendly chocolate chips or chia seeds.
8. Chia Pudding: Mix chia seeds with almond or coconut milk and let it sit to thicken. Add a splash of vanilla and a keto sweetener of choice.
9. Ham & Cream Cheese Roll-Ups: Lay out a slice of ham, spread on cream cheese, add a few asparagus or green beans, and roll!
10. Romaine Tacos: Use romaine lettuce leaves as taco shells and fill with pre-cooked chicken, guacamole, and shredded cheese.
11. Olives & Feta Bowl: Mix a variety of olives with chunks of feta cheese, a drizzle of olive oil, and some herbs.
12. Cucumber Subs: Slice a cucumber lengthwise and hollow out the seeds. Fill with deli meat, cheese, and keto condiments.
13. Cold Shrimp & Guac: Pre-cooked shrimp paired with store-bought guacamole is a divine combo.
14. Prosciutto-Wrapped Veggies: Wrap prosciutto around slices of melon or sticks of bell pepper for a salty-sweet snack.
15. Greek Salad Cup: A quick mix of cherry tomatoes, cucumber slices, olives, feta, olive oil, and oregano.
16. Coconut Yogurt Parfait: Layer keto-friendly coconut yogurt with nuts, seeds, and a few berries.
17. Keto Trail Mix: Combine nuts, seeds, coconut flakes, and keto-friendly chocolate chips for an on-the-go snack.

18. Smoked Salmon & Cream Cheese: Lay out slices of smoked salmon, spread cream cheese, sprinkle some capers, and roll.
19. Keto Muesli: Mix together seeds, nuts, and coconut flakes, and pour them over with unsweetened almond milk.
20. Veggie Dip Cups: Fill the bottom of a cup with keto-friendly dip or dressing. Add in cut veggies like bell peppers, cucumbers, and cherry tomatoes.
21. As mentioned before, sardines are an incredibly nutritious solution. If you love them, eat them straight from the tin, or pair them with keto crackers, or a prepared salad.

The beauty of zero-cook keto is that it's all about assembly, creativity, and using what you have on hand. These meal ideas are just the tip of the iceberg. With a well-stocked kitchen, your meal combinations are nearly endless. And the best part? No cooking is required! Welcome to the fuss-free keto life.

CROCKPOT KETO

Set it and Forget it: Crock Pot Keto Magic

Isn't there something magical about throwing a few ingredients into a pot in the morning and coming home to a house filled with delicious aromas and a meal ready to dive into? That's the beauty of slow cooker cooking. It's efficient, simple, and oh-so-flavorful. And let's clear the air on something: these aren't traditional "recipes" that come with a laundry list of instructions and precise measurements. Nope! These are more like *suggestions* or *inspirations*. Think of them as casual guidelines to spark your culinary creativity. The aim? To whip up something delectable without feeling tethered to a step-by-step manual.

Here are some delectable keto-friendly ideas to add to your rotation:

1. Golden Cream of Chicken Soup: chicken tenderloins, onions, celery, heavy cream, butter, simmered in chicken bone broth.
2. Tender Pork Pieces: Seasoned pork ribs ready to pile in keto street tacos, or just enjoy ala carte.
3. Tender Beef Stew: Chunked beef, radishes (a great low-carb potato substitute!), celery, beef broth, herbs, and a splash of Worcestershire sauce.
4. Garlic Butter Chicken: Whole chicken, generous dollops of butter, minced garlic, and Italian herbs.

5. Savory Lamb Shanks: Lamb shanks, beef broth, rosemary, thyme, and garlic.
6. Broccoli Cheese Soup: Broccoli florets, chicken broth, heavy cream, cheddar cheese, and seasonings.
7. Balsamic Roast Beef: Beef roast, balsamic vinegar, beef broth, and dried onion soup mix.
8. Creamy Tuscan Garlic Chicken: Chicken thighs, sun-dried tomatoes, spinach, garlic, heavy cream, and Parmesan cheese.
9. Mexican Shredded Beef: Beef chuck roast, canned diced green chilies, cumin, paprika, and beef broth.
10. Lemon Herb Salmon: Salmon fillets, lemon slices, fresh dill, butter, and chicken broth.
11. Zesty Chili Lime Chicken: Chicken breasts, lime zest, chili powder, cumin, and chicken broth.
12. Spaghetti Squash and Meatballs: Spaghetti squash (halved and seeds removed), your favorite keto meatballs, and low-carb marinara sauce.
13. Creamed Spinach Chicken: Chicken breasts, fresh spinach, cream cheese, parmesan, and garlic.
14. Buffalo Chicken Lettuce Wraps: Chicken breasts, buffalo sauce, and butter. Serve shredded in lettuce wraps with blue cheese crumbles.
15. Coconut Curry Chicken: Chicken thighs, coconut milk, curry powder, ginger, and mixed veggies like bell peppers.
16. Bacon and Mushroom Chicken: Chicken breasts, sliced mushrooms, chopped bacon, and cream of mushroom soup (keto-friendly version).

17. Eggplant Parmesan: Sliced eggplant, low-carb marinara sauce, and lots of mozzarella and parmesan cheese.
18. Italian Beef Roast: Beef roast, pepperoncini peppers, Italian seasoning, and beef broth.
19. Green Chili Pork: Pork shoulder, canned green chilies, cumin, and chicken broth.
20. Mediterranean Lamb: Lamb chunks, olives, feta cheese, rosemary, lemon juice, and chicken broth.
21. Shrimp and Sausage Gumbo: Pre-cooked sausage slices, shrimp (add during the last 30 minutes), diced tomatoes, bell peppers, celery, and Cajun seasoning.
22. Bacon-Wrapped Chicken: Chicken breasts wrapped in bacon slices, cream cheese, and your choice of seasonings.

Remember, these suggestions are templates. The beauty of slow cooker cooking is its flexibility. Feel free to experiment, swap out ingredients, and make each dish uniquely yours. One thing's for sure: you'll have a mouthwatering keto meal waiting for you at the end of the day with minimal fuss!

AIR FRYER KETO

“Almost No-Cook” Air Fryer Delights

Sometimes, we want that perfectly crispy finish without the hassle of cooking or frying. Enter the air fryer - a keto aficionado's secret weapon! Think of it as the superhero sidekick to your Grab and Go journey. It's like having the power of an oven, grill, and fryer all in one, without the long wait or the oily mess. While it might not technically be *no-cook*, it sure feels that way when meals come together so effortlessly. Here are some minimal effort, maximum flavor inspirations for your air fryer:

1. Sizzling Sausages: Whether they're fresh or frozen, throw in some sausages. In minutes, you've got a keto-friendly meal.
2. Perfect Rib Eye: Season a rib-eye steak, pop it in, and let the magic happen. It's steakhouse quality without the steakhouse price.
3. Revived Leftovers: Leftovers getting you down? Bring them back to life with a quick trip in the air fryer.
4. Winging It: Season some chicken wings and throw them in. Whether you like them spicy, tangy, or plain, they'll come out crispy every time.
5. Flash-Fried Fish: Have some frozen fish fillets? Season them, maybe add a bit of almond flour coating, and enjoy a crispy, flaky treat.
6. Bacon-Wrapped Asparagus: Wrap some fresh asparagus in bacon. It’s both fancy and fast!

7. Cheese-Stuffed Mushrooms: Remove stems, stuff with your favorite cheese, season, and let the air fryer do the work.
8. Eggplant Pizzas: Slice an eggplant, and top with some keto-friendly tomato sauce, cheese, and your favorite toppings.
9. Avocado Fries: Slice avocado, coat in almond flour, and fry them up. Creamy on the inside, crispy on the outside!
10. Zucchini or Mozzarella Sticks: Use zucchini slices or mozzarella, dip in egg, coat in Parmesan or almond flour, and air-fry until crispy.
11. Stuffed Peppers: Fill bell peppers with a mix of ground beef and cheese. It's a mini meal in a veggie vessel!
12. Shrimp Skewers: Skewer some shrimp, season, and cook. They're done before you know it!
13. Bunless Burgers: Shape your beef patties, season them, and throw them in. Perfect with some lettuce wraps and keto-friendly toppings.
14. Cauliflower Bites: Season cauliflower florets, add some buffalo sauce and enjoy a vegetarian treat.
15. Green Bean Almondine: Toss green beans in olive oil, sprinkle with slivered almonds, and cook. A classy side in no time!
16. Jalapeño Poppers: Halve jalapeños, stuff them with cream cheese, wrap them in bacon, and let them sizzle.
17. Mini Meatloaf: Shape ground beef into small patties, top with a dollop of keto ketchup, and cook. Instant mini meatloaves!
18. Salmon Patties: Mix canned salmon with an egg and some seasoning, shape them into patties, and let them crisp up.

19. Keto Nachos: Using keto-friendly tortilla chips or cheese crisps, layer with cheese and leftover meat, and melt to perfection.
20. Broccoli and Cheese Delight: Toss broccoli florets with olive oil and garlic, cook, then sprinkle with shredded cheese for the last two minutes.
21. Pork Chops: top with a pat of butter and a little Italian seasoning.

Honestly, the air fryer is a game-changer, isn't it? These aren't your grandma's complicated recipes; they are simple, straightforward inspirations. You're not slaving over a stove; you're tossing things into a basket and reclaiming your time. Give yourself a pat on the back, and enjoy these near-instant culinary delights!

SKILLET KETO

Skillet Simplicity: Quick and Easy Keto Delights

The trusty skillet—a kitchen stalwart that's perfect for the keto enthusiast who craves variety without the hassle. With its quick heating and even distribution, you can whip up a delicious keto meal in minutes. It’s not just about cooking; it’s about creating and assembling. Let’s venture into the world of skillet sensations:

1. Quick Keto Stir-Fry: Start with sliced chicken or beef. Toss in some broccoli, bell peppers, snap peas, and drizzle with a low-carb teriyaki or soy sauce. Finish with sesame seeds.
2. Creamy Garlic Shrimp: Sauté shrimp in butter with minced garlic. Stir in a splash of heavy cream and sprinkle with parsley. It’s a restaurant-worthy dish in your own kitchen!
3. Italian Sausage and Veggies: Brown Italian sausage links and toss in some zucchini, bell peppers, and a sprinkle of Italian herbs.
4. Chicken Alfredo Twist: Sauté chicken strips and pour over some keto-friendly Alfredo sauce. If you like, add spinach or broccoli. Serve over zucchini noodles for an extra twist.
5. Bacon-Wrapped Scallops: Wrap scallops in bacon strips, and sear in the skillet until crispy. Drizzle with lemon juice for a zesty finish.
6. Lemon Herb Salmon: Place salmon fillet skin-side down, and season with lemon zest, herbs, salt, and pepper. Cook until flaky. Quick, easy, and oh-so-flavorful.

7. Spicy Chorizo Eggs: Crumble chorizo in the skillet. Once browned, add beaten eggs, some diced tomatoes, and jalapeños for a spicy breakfast treat.
8. Creamy Spinach and Chicken: Brown bite-sized chicken pieces, stir in a dollop of cream cheese, a handful of spinach, and season. Watch as the spinach wilts and the sauce becomes oh-so-creamy!
9. Steak and Mushroom Delight: Sear your favorite steak cut to the desired doneness, and set aside. In the same skillet, sauté mushrooms in butter. Serve steak topped with mushrooms.
10. Pork and Green Beans: Brown some pork slices, toss in green beans, a splash of keto soy sauce, and some almond slivers.
11. Tuna Melt Revamp: Mix canned tuna with keto mayo, spread over a keto-friendly tortilla or flatbread, top with cheese, and heat until melty and crisp.
12. Cabbage and Sausage Medley: Slice up some kielbasa or any preferred sausage. Toss into the skillet with shredded cabbage, season, and enjoy a hearty, simple dish.
13. Greek Chicken Bowl: Sauté chicken cubes, then add cherry tomatoes, olives, feta cheese, and a splash of olive oil and lemon juice. An instant trip to the Mediterranean!
14. Lamb and Mint Pesto: Brown lamb chunks, and in the last few minutes of cooking, add a dollop of mint pesto. A classy dish with minimal effort!
15. Spicy Tofu Veggie Mix: For our vegetarian keto friends! Cube some firm tofu, brown in the skillet, and toss with bell peppers, broccoli, and a splash of sriracha or any spicy sauce.

16. Keto Philly Cheesesteak: Thinly slice beef, and cook quickly with sliced bell peppers, onions, and mushrooms. Top with provolone and let it melt. Enjoy as is or serve in lettuce wraps.
17. One-Pan Taco Skillet: As you beautifully described—ground beef, onions, cheese, and taco seasoning. An evergreen favorite!
18. Breakfast Sausage Skillet: Brown some breakfast sausage links, toss in spinach, and cherry tomatoes, and top with a few cracked eggs. Cover and let the eggs cook to your preference.
19. Cajun Shrimp and Sausage: Season shrimp and sausage slices with Cajun spices, then toss them into the skillet until well-cooked. A hint of the bayou in every bite!
20. Avocado Bacon Burgers: Make your beef patties and cook to your preference. Right before they're done, top with cheese, a slice of bacon, and a slice of avocado. A whole meal in one bite!
21. Spaghetti or fettuccine ala KNB: use noodles made out of konjac root for an amazing pasta experience. Create your own sugar-free tomato sauce, or feast on a cream keto alfredo. I often just put butter and garlic on these delicious pastas for a very quick serving of plant protein.
22. Bratwurst and Sauerkraut: cut up coins of bratwurst and when they're browned, pile on some sauerkraut from a jar to populate your gut microbiome with friendly bacteria.

The skillet isn't just a pan; it's an invitation to innovation. You're not slaving with complex recipes. Instead, you're assembling, creating, and tasting as you go. It's about having fun, experimenting, and finding your perfect keto blend. The next time someone tells you keto is hard, just point them to your skillet and smile!

DESSERTS

The most satisfying components of a keto regimen are these three aspects:

1. When you're in ketosis, you're never hungry.
2. When you're in ketosis, you don't have cravings.
3. When you adopt a keto lifestyle, you never need to feel deprived, so you never need to "cheat."

There are keto hacks for nearly every food you can think of, so all of the comfort foods that sabotaged your prior efforts to diet can be eaten with gusto, as long as you tweak them so that they don't spike your insulin with glucose from carbs.

The two foods I've yet to find the perfect replacement for are popcorn and French Fries, but many recipes claim they come close. However, they don't fit into our Grab and Go mentality, since they require too many steps.

There are currently more than 50,000 keto cookbooks on Amazon, and 8,000 of them are all about desserts. When you've dieted before, was your sweet tooth your downfall? Never again. If you're independently wealthy, you can buy all the dessert cookbooks and have your personal chef comb them for delectable treats to prepare for your next dinner.

However, if you're on a budget for your time *and* your money, Grab and Go desserts are all around you. No need to bake cookies or make ice cream out of strange ingredients. There are enough Grab & Go dessert options to keep you satisfied.

Note: Some people prefer to train their tastebuds away from the sweet tooth syndrome, and that is a very viable option.

Your tastebuds will definitely undergo changes with your new food choices.

Lily's chocolate candies
Keto Cookies
Keto Cake (your guests will never know the difference)
Keto ice cream
Berries by themselves
Berries with cream or whipped cream
Keto Mousse
Keto Jello
Yummy Scrummy Gummies and Caramels
Frozen berries with cream
Frozen berries with cinnamon and Chocolate Allulose
Blueberry Goo

Decadent Delights: Keto Desserts Made Easy

We've all been there: after a fulfilling meal, there's still a little space left for something sweet, a delicate ending to tie everything together. The great news for keto dieters? Indulging in these post-meal treats doesn't mean undoing all the hard work. With the keto diet, the world of desserts has been reinvented, leading to a plethora of options that will please your palate without compromising your ketosis.

Here are some more delightful options:

1. Keto Fat Bombs: These are small bite-sized treats packed with healthy fats. Made with ingredients like coconut oil, nut butters, and cocoa powder, they can provide a quick energy boost while satisfying your sweet cravings. And

the best part? They require no baking. Just mix, mold, and freeze.

2. Keto Nut Clusters: Toasted nuts like pecans or walnuts, combined with a touch of keto-friendly sweetener and perhaps a sprinkle of sea salt, then left to set. Simplicity at its best!
3. Keto Avocado Pudding: Blend ripe avocados with cocoa powder and a sweetener like stevia or erythritol. The result? A smooth, creamy, and utterly indulgent chocolate pudding.
4. Keto Protein Balls: Blend together almond or coconut flour with a protein powder of choice, a natural sweetener, and maybe a dash of unsweetened almond milk. Form into balls and chill. Perfect for a protein-packed dessert or snack!
5. Chocolate-Dipped Strawberries: Melt your favorite keto-friendly chocolate (like Lily's), dip some fresh strawberries in, and let them set in the fridge. An elegant and simple treat.
6. Keto Cheesecake Bites: Whip together some cream cheese, sweetener, and vanilla extract. Roll into balls and dip in crushed nuts or unsweetened coconut.
7. Coconut Almond Bars: Think of your favorite chocolate bar but keto-fied. Layers of desiccated coconut and almonds bound together with a rich chocolate coat.
8. Keto Tiramisu: Using almond flour for the base, layer with a rich mascarpone mix and a sprinkle of cocoa. A low-carb twist to an Italian favorite!
9. Peanut Butter Keto Cups: Just like your favorite chocolate peanut butter cups but without the sugar. Use a mold to layer keto-friendly chocolate and peanut butter. Chill to set.

10. Chia Seed Pudding: Mix chia seeds with coconut or almond milk, let them soak until they form a gel-like consistency, then top with keto-friendly fruits or a drizzle of vanilla essence.
11. Hit your favorite store for pre-made fat bombs, cookies, cakes, candies, chocolates, and ice cream. They're everywhere, even in regular grocery chains.

The keto world is full of inventive ways to keep the sweetness alive. It's about thinking outside the box, and with a bit of creativity, you can reinvent and reintroduce all your favorite desserts. The keto way of life doesn't mean cutting out the joys of indulgence; it means redefining them. So, the next time your sweet tooth starts tingling, remember there's always a keto answer waiting for you!

KETO CALENDAR

Here is a sample of what my month looks like to have a nice variety of nutrition (diversity in your gut is a good thing)!

I usually eat one or two meals a day, so I made the calendar for two meals times thirty days. If you want to go OMAD (One Meal a Day), just fit the two meals into a 60-120 minute period (1-2 hours).

Since these meals don't really have "recipes," I've shown the "assembly" on my social media. You can join me on "Keto Express" to see how quick and easy it is to assemble a keto meal in five minutes.

I doubt you would follow this calendar exactly, because you'd really want to use your groceries efficiently, so leftovers and repurposed ingredients would likely dictate your day's fare.

I personally often eat the same meal twice a day, because when you're cooking for one, sometimes you throw away more than you eat. I avoid that waste by cooking for two instead of one and spreading the same meal over one, two, three, or even four meals.

But here you have before you 60 meal plans without repetition to demonstrate to you that a month of keto could be filled with fascinating foodie adventures… never boring!

By the way, this list could go on for months without repetition if we weren't limited to "Grab and Go." I've never been bored or deprived. I love experimenting! And if you want to lose weight faster, you can forego the desserts and treats. Remember to listen to your body to be aware when it's full. These meals can be big or small, depending on your present goals of weight loss or maintenance.

Go here to see how to assemble these meals and where to find the pre-made treats to stock your pantry:

www.ketoexpress.com/menus

Remember that these menus are here to demonstrate the concept that there are sixty different proteins, sixty different veggie dishes, sixty different salads, and sixty different treats, for a total of 240 different meal options. Combine them as you like and remove anything you don't care for. I use onions a lot, even though many purists (keto police) wouldn't allow them, as they're a little bit high in carbs. I lost ninety pounds eating onions frequently, so find out what works for YOU. Combine, add, and delete to your heart's content. And remember to only eat until you're full! Use your intuition!

DAY ONE:

A. First Meal:
    1. Kansas City Butter Chicken
    2. Radish Coins with Almond Butter
    3. Broccoli Slaw with Pine Nuts
    4. Keto Chocolate Peanut Butter Cups
B. Second Meal
    1. Ham & Swiss Roll-Ups with Spicy Mayo
    2. Mini Sweet Peppers (with cream cheese if desired)
    3. Crunchy Romaine Lettuce Dippers with Keto Dressing.
    4. Keto Coffee Caramels

DAY TWO:

A. First Meal:
    1. Crock Pot Spareribs
    2. Broccoli Sprouts with Keto Dressing
    3. Seed Crackers with Cheese
    4. Keto Ice Cream

B. Second Meal
    1. Mild Sweet Italian Sausages
    2. Chopped Onions
    3. Box of Salad Greens with Olive Oil
    4. Fresh Blueberries

DAY THREE:

A. First Meal:
    1. Collard Wrap with Deli Slices
    2. Caprese Skewers
    3. Cucumber Subs
    4. Coconut Yogurt Parfait

B. Second Meal
    1. Avocado Halves Filled with Tuna Salad
    2. Greek Salad Cup
    3. Daikon Radish Sandwich Slices with Fillings
    4. Keto Trail Mix

DAY FOUR:

A. First Meal:
   1. Skillet Ground Beef with Onions
   2. Pre-prepared Cole Slaw
   3. Celery Stalks with Keto Ranch Dressing
   4. Keto Chocolate-Covered Strawberries

B. Second Meal
   1. Tortillas with Skillet Ground Beef and Cheese
   2. Avocado Slices with Salt and Pepper
   3. Spring Mix Greens with Keto Dressing
   4. Strawberries in the Snow

DAY FIVE:

B. First Meal:
   5. Garlic Butter Chicken
   6. Olives Platter
   7. 1 cup Macadamia Nuts
   8. Keto Gummy Bears

C. Second Meal
   1. Balsamic Roast Beef
   2. Bok Choy Scoopers with Keto Dressing
   3. Cucumber Boats with Seasonings
   4. Keto Caramel Ice Cream Bar

DAY SIX:

A. First Meal:
    1. Full Fat Cottage Cheese with Cracked Pepper
    2. Skillet Mushrooms with Seasonings
    3. Spring Blend Greens with MCT Oil
    4. Keto Chocolate Covered Almonds
B. Second Meal
    1. Ground Chicken with Onions (Skillet)
    2. Broccoli Sprouts with Keto Dressing
    3. ½ Cup Pistachios
    4. Keto Coconut Caramels

DAY SEVEN:

A. First Meal:
    1. Sliced Rib Eye Steak (Skillet)
    2. Charcuterie Board
    3. Broccoli slaw with pine nuts
    4. Raspberries in Cream
B. Second Meal
    1. Lemon Herb Salmon
    2. Kale with Pine Nuts and Sweet Keto Dressing
    3. Pecan Stickies (with Keto Maple Syrup)
    4. Keto Gummy Bears

DAY EIGHT:

A. First Meal:
   1. Guacamole Mash with Seed Flat "Tortillas"
   2. Romaine Lettuce Tacos
   3. Caprese Salad
   4. Keto Mini Cakes

B. Second Meal
   1. Rib Eye Steak (Air Fryer)
   2. Broccoli Florets with Keto Ranch Dressing
   3. Chopped Salad (pre-bought)
   4. Keto Chocolate Chip Cookies

DAY NINE:

A. First Meal:
   1. Creamed Spinach Chicken
   2. Air Fryer Zucchini Fries
   3. Arugula with Parmesan Shavings
   4. Keto Peppermint and White Chocolate Bar

B. Second Meal
   1. Tender Beef Stew
   2. Asparagus Wrapped in Bacon
   3. Mixed Greens with Pecans and Goat Cheese
   4. Keto Original Caramels

DAY TEN:

A. First Meal:
    1. Bacon and Mushroom Chicken
    2. Cauliflower Cheesy Mac
    3. Spinach and Mushrooms with Garlic Dressing
    4. Keto Chocolate Hazelnut Bar
B. Second Meal
    1. Eggplant Parmesan
    2. Brussel Sprouts with Creamy Butter Sauce
    3. Endive and Walnut Salad
    4. Keto Rum Balls

DAY ELEVEN:

A. First Meal:
    1. Italian Beef Roast
    2. Green Olives Platter
    3. Mixed Berry Salad with Mint
    4. Keto Cinnamon Muffins
B. Second Meal
    1. Green Chili Pork
    2. Celery (juiced at store or stalks)
    3. Radicchio with Olive Tapenade
    4. Keto Caramel Nut Chew

DAY TWELVE:

A. First Meal:
    1. Mediterranean Lamb
    2. Cabbage Sautee with Chia Seeds
    3. Asparagus and Almond Salad
    4. Chia Seed Pudding
B. Second Meal
    1. Shrimp and Sausage Gumbo
    2. Green Peppers Sliced
    3. Baby Spinach with Raspberry Vinaigrette
    4. Keto Jello

DAY THIRTEEN:

A. First Meal:
    1. Shrimp Skewers
    2. Cauliflower Florets with Ranch
    3. Radish and Cucumber Spiralized Salad
    4. Keto Magic Mousse
B. Second Meal
    1. Bacon-Wrapped Chicken Breasts
    2. Air Fryer Green Bean Fries
    3. Cobb Salad with Keto Ranch
    4. Blueberry Goo

DAY FOURTEEN:

A. First Meal:
    1. Sizzling Sausages
    2. Red Peppers with Blue Cheese
    3. Seaweed Salad with Sesame Dressing
    4. Keto Fat Bombs (Bought or Pre-Made)
B. Second Meal
    1. Chicken Wings with Honey Mustard Dressing
    2. Air Fryer Jicama Fries
    3. Grilled Shrimp and Avocado Salad with Cilantro Lime Dressing
    4. Keto Avocado Pudding

DAY FIFTEEN:

A. First Meal:
    1. Eggplant Pizza
    2. Cauliflower Bites
    3. Warm Bacon and Brussels sprouts Salad
    4. Keto Cheesecake Bites
B. Second Meal
    1. Stuffed Bell Peppers
    2. Jalapeno Poppers
    3. Kalamata Olive and Cherry Tomato Salad with Fresh Basil
    4. Chocolate Fruit Fondue

DAY SIXTEEN:

A. First Meal:
    1. Bunless Burger
    2. Daikon Radish Mini PB&J Finger Sandwiches
    3. Seared Tuna Salad with Wasabi Mayo and Sesame Seeds
    4. Keto Brownies

B. Second Meal
    1. Meatloaf
    2. Asparagus Spears with Parmesan Sprinkle
    3. Iceberg Wedge Salad
    4. Keto Cups

DAY SEVENTEEN:

A. First Meal:
    1. Pork Chops
    2. Cauliflower Rice with Scallions
    3. Smoked Salmon and Dill Salad over Mixed Greens
    4. Coconut Flake Fat Bombs

B. Second Meal
    1. Keto Stir Fry
    2. Crispy Roasted Brussel Sprouts
    3. Leaf Lettuce with Arugula and Sprouts
    4. Frozen Cream Whips (pre-made by you)

DAY EIGHTEEN:

A. First Meal:
    1. Italian Sausage with Onions and Peppers
    2. Crudites with Low-Carb Dip
    3. Boston Lettuce with Walnuts and Keto Dressing
    4. Keto Almond Dark Chocolate Bar
B. Second Meal
    1. Chicken Pasta Alfredo
    2. Cauliflower Mashed Potatoes
    3. Bibb Lettuce with Sliced Almonds and Keto Dressing
    4. Keto Chocolate Covered Peanuts

DAY NINETEEN:

A. First Meal:
    1. Bacon-Wrapped Scallops
    2. Cheese Crisp Crackers with Salami Slices
    3. Mesclun Mix with Strawberries
    4. Keto Chocolate Nibs (handful)
B. Second Meal
    1. Lemon Herb Salmon
    2. Stuffed Cherry Tomatoes with Pesto and Parmesan
    3. Watercress Salad
    4. Keto Butterscotch Nibs (handful)

DAY TWENTY:

A. First Meal:
   1. Spicy Chorizo Eggs
   2. Roasted Cauliflower Steaks with Garlic Butter
   3. Keto Caesar Salad
   4. Keto White Chocolate Nibs (handful)

B. Second Meal
   1. Steak and Mushroom Delight
   2. Chilled Cucumber Soup with Fresh Herbs
   3. Spinach Salad with Bacon and Hard-Boiled Eggs
   4. Keto Caramel Nibs (Handful)

DAY TWENTY-ONE:

A. First Meal:
   1. Pork and Green Beans
   2. Keto Broccoli and Cheddar Soup
   3. BLT Salad
   4. Keto Pumpkin Spice Nibs (handful)

B. Second Meal
   1. Tuna Melt Revamp
   2. Buttery Lemon-Garlic Brussel Sprouts
   3. Mixed Greens with Champagne Vinaigrette
   4. Keto Chocolate Mint Nibs (handful)

DAY TWENTY-TWO:

A. First Meal:
   1. Bratwurst and Cabbage
   2. Turnip Fries with Keto Ketchup
   3. Lettuce and Avocado with Keto Lime Dressing
   4. Keto Chocolate Covered Caramels

B. Second Meal
   1. Greek Chicken Bowl
   2. Cheesy Cauliflower Frittata
   3. Swiss Chard with Toasted Walnuts
   4. Keto Hazelnut Bar

DAY TWENTY-THREE:

A. First Meal:
   1. Lamb Mint Pesto
   2. Spicy Tofu Veggie Mix
   3. Keto Waldorf Salad
   4. Mocha Hot Coca Extreme Dark Chocolate Bar

B. Second Meal
   1. Keto Philly Cheesesteak
   2. Keto Ratatouille with Fresh Basil
   3. Sardine Salad
   4. Keto Strawberry Ice Cream with Strawberries

DAY TWENTY-FOUR:

A. First Meal:
   1. One Pan Taco Skillet
   2. Zucchini Ribbons Salad with Olive Oils and Lemon Vinaigrette
   3. Greek Salad
   4. Keto Salted Caramel Milk Chocolate Bar

B. Second Meal
   1. Breakfast Sausage Skillet
   2. Stuffed Bell Peppers with Ground Beef and Cheese
   3. Sprouts Medley with Southwest Dressing
   4. Keto Sea Salt Extra Dark Chocolate Bar

TWENTY-FIVE:

A. First Meal:
   1. Avocado Bacon Burger
   2. Roasted Eggplant Slices with Olive Tapenade
   3. Creamy Cucumber Salad
   4. Keto Ice Cream Sandwich

B. Second Meal
   1. Fettucine with Sauce (Alfredo, Tomato, Garlic)
   2. Spaghetti Squash with Keto Alfredo Sauce
   3. Cauliflower Potato Salad
   4. Keto Natural Vanilla Ice Cream with Toppings

5.

DAY TWENTY-SIX:

A. First Meal:
   1. Bratwurst and Sauerkraut
   2. Brussel Sprouts with Creamy Butter Sauce
   3. Warm Kale with Dijon
   4. Keto Mint Chip Ice Cream

B. Second Meal
   1. Sesame Seared Ahi Tuna with Keto Soy Sauce
   2. Spinach and Artichoke Dip Cups
   3. Zucchini, Spring Greens, and Walnuts
   4. Keto Triple Chocolate Ice Cream

TWENTY-SEVEN:

A. First Meal:
   1. Chopped Chicken Breast Veggie Medley
   2. Riced Cauliflower with Pesto and Sun-Dried Tomatoes
   3. Cabbage Salad
   4. Keto Vanilla Crunch Ice Cream Bar

B. Second Meal
   1. Skillet Pizza
   2. Buttery Lemon Asparagus Spears
   3. Chopped Veggie Salad
   4. Keto Sea Salt Caramel Crunch Ice Cream Bar

TWENTY-EIGHT:

A. First Meal:
    1. Liver and Onions
    2. Zucchini and Yellow Squash Medley
    3. Broccoli Salad with Bacon
    4. Keto Munk Pack Seed Bars
B. Second Meal
    1. Beef Stroganoff over Konjac Noodles
    2. Sauteed Kale with Garlic and Red Pepper Flakes
    3. Daikon Radish Salad
    4. Keto Sour Gummy Worms

DAY TWENTY-NINE:

A. First Meal:
    1. Lobster Tails with Butter Sauce
    2. Roasted Broccoli with Parmesan and Almonds
    3. Veggie Slaw with Chia Seeds
    4. Blackberry Mash
B. Second Meal
    1. Seared Scallops with Scallion Relish
    2. Zucchini Zoodles Salad with Avocado Dressing
    3. Romaine Fingers with Egg Salad
    4. Keto Chocolate Swiss Roll

DAY THIRTY:

A. First Meal:
    1. Cold Crab with Dijon Sauce
    2. Fried Okra Bites
    3. Iceberg Lettuce Skinny Wedges with Dip
    4. Keto Toffee Chocolate Squares
B. Second Meal
    1. Shrimp Scampi
    2. Sauteed Spinach
    3. Prepackaged Southwest Salad with Keto Dressing
    4. Keto Blueberry Lemon Bundt Cake

TO FIND THE INSTRUCTIONS FOR MENU ITEMS ONLINE GO TO www.KNBsKetoExpress.com/menus

The alphabetical lists that follow are for your convenience in finding the items online.

PROTEIN PORTIONS (ALPHABETICAL)

Avocado Bacon Burger
Avocado Halves with Tuna Salad
Liver and Onions
Bacon and Mushroom Chicken
Bacon-Wrapped Chicken Breasts
Bacon-Wrapped Scallops
Balsamic Roast Beef
Beef Stroganoff Over Konjac Noodles
Bratwurst and Cabbage
Bratwurst and Sauerkraut
Breakfast Sausage Skillet
Bunless Burger
Chicken Pasta Alfredo
Chicken Wings with Honey Mustard Dressing
Chopped Chicken Breast Veggie Medley
Cold Crab with Dijon Sauce
Collar Wrap with Deli Slices
Creamed Spinach Chicken
Crock Pot Spareribs
Eggplant Parmesan
Eggplant Pizza
Fettucine with Choice of Sauce
Full Fat Cottage Cheese with Cracked Pepper
Garlic Butter Chicken
Greek Chicken Bowl
Green Chili Pork
Ground Chicken with Onions
Guacamole Mash with Seed Flat "Tortillas"

Ham & Swiss Roll-Ups with Spicy Mayo
Italian Beef Roast
Italian Sausage with Onions and Peppers
Kansas City Butter Chicken
Keto Stir Fry
Lamb Mint Pesto
Lemon Herb Salmon
Lemon Herb Salmon
Lobster Tails with Butter Sauce
Meatloaf
Mild Sweet Italian Sausages
One Pan Taco Skillet
Philly Cheesesteak
Mediterranean Lamb
Pork and Green Beans
Pork Chops
Rib Eye Steak (Air Fryer)
Seared Scallops with Scallion Relish
Sesame Seared Ahi Tuna with Keto Soy Sauce
Shrimp and Sausage Gumbo
Shrimp Scampi
Shrimp Skewers
Sizzling Sausages
Skillet Ground Beef and Onions
Skillet Pizza
Sliced Rib Eye Steak (Skillet)
Spicy Chorizo Eggs
Steak and Mushroom Delight
Stuffed Bell Peppers
Tender Beef Stew
Tortillas with Skillet Ground Beef and Cheese

VEGGIE PORTIONS
(ALPHABETICAL)

Air Fryer Green Bean Fries
Air Fryer Jicama Fries
Air Fryer Zucchini Fries
Asparagus Spears with Parmesan Sprinkle
Asparagus Wrapped in Bacon
Avocado Slices with Salt and Pepper
Bok Choy Scoopers and Keto Dressing
Broccoli Florets with Keto Ranch
Broccoli Sprouts with Keto Dressing
Broccoli Sprouts with MCT Oil and Sweet Mustard
Brussel Sprouts Roasted with Keto Balsamic Vinegar
Brussels sprouts with Creamy Butter Sauce
Buttery Lemon Asparagus Spears
Buttery Lemon-Garlic Brussels Sprouts
Cabbage Sautee with Chia Seeds
Caprese Skewers
Cauliflower Bites
Cauliflower Cheesy Mac
Cauliflower Florets with Ranch
Cauliflower Mashed "Potatoes"
Cauliflower Rice with Scallions
Celery (Juiced at the Store or Stalks)
Charcuterie Board
Cheese Crisp Crackers and Salami Slices
Chilled Cucumber Soup with Fresh Herbs
Chopped Onions
Crispy Roasted Brussels sprouts

Crudites with Low-Carb Dip
Daikon Radish Mini PB&J Finger Sandwiches
Fried Okra Bites
Greek Salad Cup
Green Olives Platter
Green Pepper Slices
Jalapeno Poppers
Kale with Pine Nuts and Sweet Keto Dressing
Keto Broccoli and Cheddar Soup
Keto Ratatouille with Fresh Basil
Mini Sweet Peppers with Cream Cheese
Olives Platter
Pre-Prepared Cole Slaw
Radish Coins with Almond Butter
Ramine Lettuce Tacos
Red Peppers with Blue Cheese
Riced Cauliflower with Pesto and Sun-dried Tomatoes
Roasted Broccoli with Parmesan and Almonds
Roasted Cauliflower Steaks with Garlic Butter
Roasted Eggplant Slices with Olive Tapenade
Sautéed Kale with Garlic and Red Pepper Flakes
Spaghetti Squash with Keto Alfredo Sauce
Spicy Tofu Veggie Mix
Spinach and Artichoke Dip Cups
Stuffed Bell Peppers with Ground Beef and Cheese
Stuffed Cherry Tomatoes with Pesto, Parmesan
Stuffed Portobello Mushrooms with Spinach and Ricotta
Turnip Fries with Keto Ketchup
Turnip Fries with Keto Ketchup

Zucchini and Yellow Squash Medley
Zucchini Noodle "Zoodles" Salad with Avocado Dressing

SALAD PORTIONS (ALPHABETICAL)

Arugula with Parmesan Shavings
Asparagus and Almond Salad
Baby Spinach with Raspberry Vinaigrette
Bibb Lettuce with Sliced Almonds
BLT Salad
Boston Lettuce with Walnuts
Box of Greens with Olive Oil
Broccoli Salad with bacon
Broccoli Slaw with Pine Nuts
Cabbage Salad
Caprese Salad
Cauliflower Potato Salad
Celery Stalks and Keto Ranch
Chopped Salad (Store-bought)
Cobb Salad with Keto Ranch Dressing
Creamy Cucumber Salad
Crunchy Romaine Dippers
Cucumber Subs
Daikon Radish Salad
Daikon Radish Sandwich Slices
Endive and Walnut Salad
Greek Salad

Grilled Shrimp and Avocado Salad, Cilantro Lime
Iceberg Lettuce Skinny Wedges with Dip
Iceberg Wedge Salad
Kalamata Olive and Cherry Tomato with Basil
Keto Caesar Salad
Keto Waldorf Salad
Mesclun Mix with Strawberries
Mixed Berry Salad with Mint
Mixed Greens with Pecans and Goat Cheese
Radicchio with Olive Tapenade
Radish and Cucumber Spiralized Salad
Romaine Fingers with Egg Salad
Sardine Salad
Seared Tuna Salad with Wasabi May
Seaweed Salad with Sesame Dressing
Smoked Salmon and Dill over Mixed Greens
Southwest Salad
Spinach and Mushroom, Garlic Dressing
Spinach Salad with Bacon and Hard Boilled Eggs
Spring Blend Greens with MCT Oil
Spring Mix Greens with Keto Dressing
Sprouts Medley with Southwest Dressing
Swiss Chard with Toasted Walnuts
Veggie Slaw with Chia Seeds
Warm Bacon and Brussels Sprouts Salad
Warm Kale with Dijon Sauce
Watercress Salad
Zucchini, Spring Greens and Walnuts

DESSERT PORTIONS
(ALPHABETICAL)

Blackberry Mash
Blueberry Goo
Chia Seed Pudding
Chocolate Fruit Fondue
Coconut Flake Fat Bombs
Coconut Yogurt Parfait
Fresh Blueberries
Frozen Cream Whips (pre-made by YOU)
Keto "Munk Pack" Seed Bar
Keto Almond Dark Chocolate Bar
Keto Avocado Pudding
Keto Blueberry Lemon Bundt Cake
Keto Brownies
Keto Butterscotch Nibs (Handful)
Keto Caramel Ice Cream Bar
Keto Caramel Nibs (Handful)
Keto Caramel Nut Chew
Keto Cheesecake Bites
Keto Chocolate Cake
Keto Chocolate Chip Cookies
Keto Chocolate Chip Vanilla Ice Cream Sandwich
Keto Chocolate Covered Almonds
Keto Chocolate Covered Caramels
Keto Chocolate Covered Peanuts
Keto Chocolate Mint Nibs (Handful)
Keto Chocolate Nibs (Handful)
Keto Chocolate Peanut Butter Cups
Keto Peppermint and White Chocolate Bars

Keto Chocolate Hazelnut Bars
Keto Chocolate Swiss Roll
Keto Chocolate-Covered Strawberries
Keto Cinnamon Muffins
Keto Coconut Caramels
Keto Coffee Caramels
Keto Cups
Keto Fat Bombs (Bought or Pre-Made)
Keto Gummy Bears
Keto Hazelnut Bar
Keto Ice Cream
Keto Jello
Keto M&M Style Hard Candies
Keto Magic Mousse
Keto Mini Cakes
Keto Mint Chip Ice Cream
Keto Mocha Hot Cocoa Extreme Dark Bar
Keto Natural Vanilla Ice Cream with Toppings
Keto Original Caramels
Keto Pumpkin Spice Nibs (Handful)
Keto Rum Balls
Keto Salted Caramel Milk Chocolate Bar
Keto Sea Sale Caramel Crunch Ice Cream Bar
Keto Sea Salt Extra Dark Chocolate Bar
Keto Sour Gummy Worms
Keto Toffee Chocolate Squares
Keto Trail Mix
Keto Triple Chocolate Ice Cream
Keto Vanilla Crunch Ice Cream Bar
Keto White Chocolate Nibs (Handful)
Peppermint White Chocolate Bar

Raspberries in Cream
Strawberries in the Snow

CONCLUSION

From Keto Beginnings to Super Senior Thriving

Congratulations on making it through this guide. By now, you've explored many ways to simplify and enjoy the keto lifestyle, even on your busiest days. However, remember that the keto journey is more than just recipes and grab-and-go solutions. It's a mindset shift, a commitment to healthier living, and a bridge to holistic wellness.

The beautiful thing about a journey is that there's always a next step, a new horizon. You've set the foundation for your keto lifestyle, but I encourage you not to stop here. Use this newfound knowledge and energy to further enhance your life in other areas.

As you continue to navigate your health and wellness journey, I'd love to personally invite you to join me in a more intimate and connected space - a friendly coaching relationship. Together, we can delve deeper into your unique needs, challenges, and aspirations, crafting a tailored approach that aligns perfectly with your lifestyle and goals.

As life progresses, our needs change. The hurdles faced by a sprightly 25-year-old differ vastly from those of a vibrant 65-year-old. This progression led me to establish the **SUPER SENIOR** world - a space dedicated to thriving in our golden years. Whether you're approaching these years or are already in the midst of them, the SUPER SENIOR series is an extension of this journey we've started together.

By embracing the keto lifestyle, you've shown that you're not only committed to your best health but also open to exploration and learning. The SUPER SENIOR world offers not just dietary insights but also strategies to maintain mental agility, physical fitness, and a rich, fulfilling life as we age gracefully.
In conclusion, remember: our wellness journey never truly ends.

Each day presents new opportunities, challenges, and joys. Whether you choose to step into the coaching arena or immerse yourself in the SUPER SENIOR series next, know that you are not alone. Let's continue to grow, learn, and thrive together, celebrating every milestone and facing every challenge side by side. Thank you for allowing me to guide you through this page of your life. Here's to many more chapters, each richer, brighter, and more fulfilling than the last.

RESOURCES

Internet Opinion Leaders:
Dr. Eric Berg
Dr. Jason Fung
Thomas DeLauer
Vinnie Tortorich
Dr. Annette Bosworth (Dr. Boz)
Dr. Josh Axe
Dr. Nicholas Zyrowski
Dr. Mindy Pelz
Dr. Mark Hyman
Dr. Ken Berry

Documentaries:
FAT: A Documentary
Magic Pill
Real Skinny on Fat
Rotten
What the Health
The Big Lie
American Addict
Is Sugar the New Fat?
Why Are We Fat?
Diet Fiction
Fat v Carbs

Books:
The Healthy Keto Plan, Dr. Eric Berg
Any Way You Can, Dr. Annette Bosworth
Healthy Keto & Intermittent Fasting, A Simple Overview, Dr. Eric Berg
Dr. Colbert's Keto Zone Diet, Dr. Don Colbert
The Keto Reset Diet: Reboot Your Metabolism in 21 Days and Burn Fat Forever, by Mark Sisson.
Fat for Fuel, Dr. Joseph Mercola
Fast Like a Girl, Dr. Mindy Pelzz

ABOUT THE AUTHOR

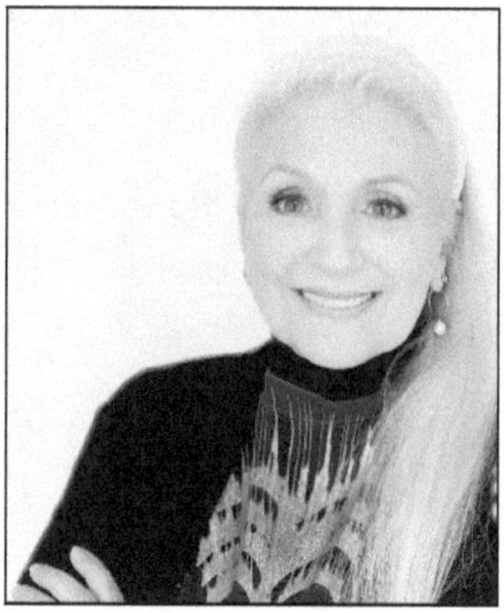

For over five decades, Karen Nelson Bell ("KNB") has graced stages and screens, captivating audiences with her talents as a singer, pianist, and dynamic force in musical direction and production. She's not just a master in the arts; in 2007, she soared to Amazon best-seller status with her expertise in real estate investing.

However, being in the limelight came with its shadows. Throughout her career, Karen faced unrelenting scrutiny and judgment about her weight. At the tender age of sixteen, she stepped onto the all-too-familiar dieting roller coaster, experiencing the highs and lows that resonate with many who've grappled with weight concerns.

Karen doesn't don a doctor's white coat, nor does she claim to be a diet aficionado or a science whiz. Instead, she wears her heart on her sleeve, generously sharing the strategies that have paved her way to success, be it in melodies, the marketplace, or managing weight.

With a genuine desire to uplift and inspire, Karen extends an invitation: embark on this journey with her and discover the unique path that leads to the best version of yourself.

OTHER BOOKS BY KNB

KNB's Keto Calendar
Nothing Down for Women
Bedtime Stories for Peaceful Sleep
Coming Soon:

- Super Senior (The Series)
- Saving America
- In Praise of Kindness
- One Heart for Harmony

ACKNOWLEDGEMENTS

The acknowledgment section of a book lets the author thank all the people without whom the book wouldn't see the light of day. I would never have even thought of writing Keto Express if it weren't for Lynn Simington.

Lynn told me that she needed to reshape her daily routines, including cleaning up her eating habits. She was interested in learning more about keto. However, she didn't have time to prepare complicated meals and menus. She really didn't even have time to learn what to do to embrace the keto lifestyle. It all seemed too complicated.

Well, my specialty as an author has always been to make things simple, from the time I entered the world as a writer with the nickname "The 5-Minute Mentor." Who has time for anything these days? I knew the moment that the phone call with Lynn ended that I would write a new keto book to handle Lynn's problem because it was *everyone's* problem. Mine too.

Thank you, Lynn, for the inspiration.

And if it weren't for the other authors who have inspired me, I would have never been able to refine my own keto lifestyle. My first and foremost mentor was renowned health guru Dr. Eric Berg. I also did a deep dive with Doctors Mindy Peltz and Annette Bosworth (Dr. Boz).

Add in Dr. Jason Fung on the subject of fasting, and non-doctor nutrition researcher Thomas DeLauer, and you can retrace my steps in learning the fascinating dynamics of keto along with intermittent fasting.

Let me also acknowledge my fellow keto buddies for sharing their stories and journeys with me. I'm a hope-a-holic, and I pray that you, the reader, will share your keto adventures with me too!

Made in United States
Troutdale, OR
11/03/2026

56844437R00070